Cancer Pain Relief

A Practical Manual

Edited by:

F. DE CONNO, MD
Istituto Nazionale per lo Studio
e la Cura dei Tumori
Milan, Italy

K. FOLEY, MD
Memorial Sloan Kettering
New York, New York, U.S.A.

Editorial Board:

DEREK DOYLE, MD
St. Columba's Hospice
Edinburgh, Great Britain

CARL JOHAN FURST
Stockholms Sjukhem
Stockholm, Sweden

JOHAN MENTEN, MD
University Hospital
Leuven, Belgium

H. PICHLMAIER, MD
Klinik und Poliklinik für Chirurgie
Köln, Germany

PHILIPPE POULAIN, MD
Institut Gustave Roussy
Villejuif-Cedex, France

CHIARA TICOZZI, MD
Istituto Nazionale per lo Studio
e la Cura dei Tumori
Milan, Italy

PAT WEBB
Trinity Hospice
London, Great Britain

SPRINGER SCIENCE+BUSINESS MEDIA, B.V.

Library of Congress Cataloging-in-Publication Data

Cancer pain relief. A practical manual / edited by F. De Conno, K.
Foley.
      p.   cm.
   Includes index.
   ISBN 978-0-7923-3590-0   ISBN 978-94-011-0099-1 (eBook)
   DOI 10.1007/978-94-011-0099-1
   1. Cancer pain--Treatment.   I. De Conno, F.   II. Foley, Kathleen
M., 1944-   .
   [DNLM: 1. Neoplasms--complications.   2. Pain, Intractable--drug
therapy.   3. Analgesics, Opioid--pharmacology.   QZ 200 P8946 1995]
RC262.P73   1995
616.99'4--dc20
DNLM/DLC
for Library of Congress   95-4898

ISBN 978-0-7923-3590-0

Cancer Pain Relief

Contents

Foreword

Pain in oncology, and especially in patients with advanced disease, is an essential issue which cannot be overlooked.

Today, pain is worldwide recognised as a very complex symptom which includes different aspects such as somatic, spiritual, social and psychological pain.

Practical and scientific knowledge of pain in cancer should be part of the pre and post training of general practioners and oncologists.

This manual reflects the opinion of different authors, contributors to pain clinic. These guidelines cover all different aspects of cancer pain. It responds to a need for information, education and training in the field of diagnosis and treatment of cancer pain. The reader will find useful information and suggestions as how to diagnose and treat pain from a pharmacological, surgical and psychosocial point of view.

Pain therapy is a very important part of quality of life; due to its relevance, we think that this manual will be a useful tool for all health professionals, and we are grateful to Drs. K. Foley and F. De Conno for their generous contribution in making this effort successful.

Alberto Costa
Director
European School of Oncology

Acknowledgements

The European School of Oncology wishes to acknowledge Janssen Pharmaceutica for an educational grant for the sponsorship of this manual.

Pain – definitions, classification and causes

The definition of pain most widely accepted is that given by the International Association for the Study of Pain (IASP) and according to which, pain is a sensory and emotional experience associated with actual or potential tissue damage, or described in terms of such damage. Pain is always subjective: pain is what the patient says hurts. This definition underlines the emotional dimension of pain and describes it both as a sensation (conscious awareness of a noxious stimulus) and as an emotional experience (intense feelings of displeasure resulting in a set of behaviours). The origin of physical pain always comes from a physical stimulus and is always modified by the mind. Other definitions stress the variety of different factors which may cause or aggravate a person's pain.

The distinction between acute and chronic pain is of great importance in the management of patients with advanced cancer, because each requires a different approach to treatment.

Acute pain is usually due to a definable nociceptive cause; its onset is recognisable and its duration is limited and predictable. It may be accompanied by anxiety and clinical signs of sympathetic overactivity: tachycardia, tachypnoea, hypertension, sweating, pupillary dilatation and pallor are characteristic signs of a suffering patient. The psychological impact of acute pain anxiety responds to reassurance that the pain will resolve with time. However, where acute pain indicates progression of cancer (or is thought to by the patient), it may be associated with depression and withdrawal more commonly seen with chronic pain. Patients who are aware that their pain is temporary have a more positive attitude.

Chronic pain results from a chronic pathological process. It has a gradual or ill-defined onset, continues unabated and may become progressively more severe. Patients appear depressed and withdrawn and, as there are usually no signs of sympathetic overactivity, sometimes they seem to be free of pain. These patients have symptoms of depression, lethargy, apathy, anorexia and insomnia. Personality changes may occur, due to progressive alterations in lifestyle and functional ability. For patients with chronic pain related to cancer, pain is usually regarded as having definite negative implications with regard to their prognosis and life expectancy. Chronic pain related to cancer requires treatment of the underlying disease where possible, regular use of analgesics to control pain symptoms and to prevent pain recurrence, as well as psychological and social supportive care as therapy. Successful treatment is often associated with a dramatic improvement in the patient's well-being.

Establishing the dividing line between acute and chronic pain is not simple: for non-malignant pain, chronic pain is said to exist if it persists longer than the expected healing time of the pathology in question; for patients with malignant cancer, and in the absence of an acute illness, pain lasting more than three months should be considered as chronic.

Nociceptive pain is produced by stimulation of specific sensory receptors or nociceptors located in the tissues. Somatic pain from the skin and superficial structures is usually well localised and described as aching, sharp, throbbing or pressure-like. Visceral pain from deeper structures is less well localised and felt over a larger area and is often referred to cutaneous areas. It may be described as a deep aching or throbbing pain and may become sharp if organ capsules are involved; obstruction of hollow viscera causes gnawing or colicky pain.

Neuropathic pain is caused by peripheral or central nervous system injury. If the central nervous system is involved it is considered as central pain and non-dermatomal in distribution, whereas pain from peripheral nerve lesions (or deafferentation pain) is dermatomal in distribution. Pain occurs because the injured nerves react abnormally to stimuli or discharge spontaneously; it is described as a burning, a stinging or stabbing pain. Pain from damaged sympathetic nerves is similar to deafferentation pain and is associated with vasomotor signs. This kind of pain responds poorly to both opioids and non-opioids but may be relieved by regional sympathetic nerve block.

Psychogenic pain does not stem from a physical basis; whilst there is no doubt that psychological factors are quite important, pure psychogenic pain is very rare, except in some patients with a prior history of psychiatric illness.

The majority of pains in patients with cancer are due to direct tumour involvement, but they may also be due to treatment or due to the debilitating effects of advancing disease, or may be unrelated to the cancer or treatment.

Pain caused by tumour infiltration

Bone metastases are the most frequent cause of pain directly attributable to cancer. They cause local pain and tenderness. The pain is constant, described as aching or annoying, and is aggrav-

ated by movement. Pain can suddenly become more intense in the event of a pathological fracture. Bone metastases can cause pain by local bone destruction, infiltration of surrounding tissues, secondary muscle spasm, or by compression of neurological structures. Compression and infiltration of a peripheral nerve may be first manifested as a dull ache, progressing to a constant superficial burning pain in the area of sensory loss, sometimes associated with hyperaesthesia, dysaesthesia and stabbing pain. For example, infiltration of the brachial plexus will cause pain and sensory loss in the C5–T1 distribution as well as motor signs in the upper limb; infiltration of the lumbar plexus will produce sensory symptoms, including pain, accompanied by motor weakness of the affected muscles.

Soft tissue infiltration causes pain because of local tissue destruction and by infiltration of pain-sensitive tissues such as fasciae or the periosteum. The pain is usually dull and aching. This could be due to compression or infiltration of nerves and vessels. Infiltration of the skin and mucous membranes is sometimes aggravated by secondary infection. Infiltration of hollow viscera causes dull pain that is poorly localised and may sharpen and become more severe if organ capsules are involved.

Pain caused by treatment

Painful neuropathy may occur after any surgical procedures particularly following thoracotomy, mastectomy or neck dissection. The pain develops several months following the procedure and is a deep continuous dull ache with intermittent stabbing pain or a continuous burning dysaesthesia with hyperaesthesia.

Similarly, patients undergoing amputation can develop a constant aching or burning pain in the stump or in the phantom limb.

Chemotherapy causes painful mucositis and phlebitis; tissue necrosis may occur if there is extravasation of drugs into the tissues. Painful neuropathy may develop after treatment with vinca alkaloids; if corticosteroids are suddenly withdrawn, painful myalgia and arthralgia may occur.

Radiation fibrosis with secondary nerve compression involving either the brachial or lumbosacral plexus causes painful neuropathy, starting usually after at least one year. Radiotherapy also produces painful mucositis (including cystitis), and myelopathy, with a delay of more than six months, may occur if the spinal cord has been radiated by a dose higher than spinal cord tolerance.

Pain related to debilitating disease

In advanced cancer, a small proportion of the pain relates directly to the effects of the debilitating disease. Myofascial pain originates from a muscle and its surrounding fascia and it is characterised by a localised trigger point, the stimulation of which produces pain that radiates in a non-dermatomal manner.

Pain unrelated to cancer or treatment

About one-fifth of pains reported by cancer patients are due to factors other than cancer or its therapy, for example various forms of arthritis, or pain due to ischaemic heart disease and peripheral vascular disease.

Factors that modify the perception of pain – the concept of clinical pain

The perception of pain is subject to modification by many different factors: physical, psychological, social, cultural and spiritual. Dame Cicely Saunders introduced the concept of "Total Pain", being the sum of these factors, in order to emphasise the complex nature of pain and the need to consider it as a whole, so that its treatment may be successful. The concept of Total Pain should be distinguished from that of Total Suffering, which in reality is the sum of the effects of the various causes of suffering, of which pain is only one. The other causes of suffering may simultaneously modify the perception of pain, resulting in Clinical Pain. The term Clinical Pain is used here to describe the pain as felt by the patient, incorporating all the modifying effects from the other causes of potential suffering. Physical pain can be modified by a number of different factors related to the various causes of potential suffering that result in the final Clinical Pain. These modifying factors may have either a positive or negative effect on the perception of pain, causing either exacerbation or amelioration, even though in clinical practice this second possibility is generally the one most frequently seen, it is also not uncommon to see patients who complain of much less pain than might be expected from their medical situation. In some circumstances the patient's pain is wholly attributable to other causes of suffering. The Clinical Pain represents what the patient says it is and it must be treated.

These various modifying factors are aetiologically interrelated with pain and therefore sometimes create a vicious circle. Factors related to the patient's physical pain may modify the perception of pain: for example severe or progressive pain, pain at multiple or an increasing number of sites or poor pain management or significant limitation of activity can all aggravate the perception of pain; contrasting situations may ameliorate pain. The effect of good management of all chronic pain on the perception of future pain cannot be overestimated.

The presence of other physical symptoms such as persistent cough, vomiting and prolonged hiccups may aggravate the perception of pain. The same is also to be considered for psychological problems (anxiety, depression) as well as for social difficulties. The concept of clinical pain depicts the dynamic interaction that occurs between the various causes of suffering and underlines the difference between pain and suffering; the important clinical corollary is that all problems related to other causes of suffering must be assessed and treated if pain control is to be successful.

Initial pain assessment

The initial pain assessment should focus on identifying the cause of the pain and developing a pain management plan. Subsequent assessments should evaluate the effectiveness of the plan and, if pain is unrelieved, bring about any necessary changes. The initial evaluation of pain should include an accurate detailed history, including an assessment of the pain intensity and character, a physical examination with particular emphasis on the neurologic examination, a psychosocial assessment and an appropriate diagnostic workup to determine the cause of the pain.

Attention to detail is important: a delayed diagnosis of spinal cord compression can result in increased morbidity with resultant paraplegia. The patient's self-report should be the primary source of assessment. This is best achieved by encouraging the patient to tell their own story – all dimensions of pain can then be ascertained. In addition it may be preferable to use brief easy-to-use assessment tools. The ones most commonly used are:

– Pain Intensity Scale;
– Numeric pain Intensity Scale;
– Visual Analog Scale (VAS); and
– Body Charts.

It is necessary to elicit information regarding the influence pain has on the patient's daily activities, including both work and recreational activities, sleep patterns, mobility, appetite and sexual functioning.

A psychosocial assessment should emphasise the effect of pain on both patients and their families. Appropriate diagnostic tests should be performed to determine the cause of the pain and the extent of disease; it is important to correlate the results of these studies with physical and neurological findings. It is necessary to mention that pain may be the first sign of tumour recurrence or progression, even before changes are evident in imaging studies.

Pain assessment during treatment

Pain should be assessed and documented at regular intervals after beginning the treatment plan: suitable intervals are necessary to document the pharmacological effect. Occasionally, discrepancies between behaviours and a patient's self-report of his pain may occur; these may result from several factors, including the effectiveness of the patient's coping skills or his inability to communicate adequately for whatever reason. In the assessment of pain, the role of team members: doctors, nurses, physiotherapists, psychologists, social workers, etc. is of great importance from the very beginning and throughout the period of treatment.

Assessment of common cancer pain syndromes

1. Abdominal pain

Abdominal pain due to abdominal tumours can be caused by different pathophysiologies such as: upper abdominal pains due to, liver metastases (liver capsule pain), gastrointestinal obstruction, peritoneal carcinomatosis, pancreatic cancer syndromes; lower abdominal and pelvic pains due to rectal, bladder, vaginal and perineal tumour infiltration.

2. Acute and postherpetic neuralgia

Varicella-zoster virus reactivation is more likely to occur in patients with cancer because of their immunosuppression. The virus may cause both acute and chronic pain. The infection is characterised by a burning aching pain with stabbing pain in areas with skin lesions that are usually hypoaesthesic. In acute phases antiviral therapies in combination with analgesics are recommended, whereas for postherpetic neuralgia therapies for neuropathic pain are used. Nerve block seems to reduce pain intensity, shorten the acute episode and may prevent the emergence of postherpetic neuralgia. There is certainly evidence that TENS can relieve postherpetic neuralgia.

3. Bone metastases

Cancers of the breast, prostate, lung and multiple myeloma account for a large majority of bone metastases. The most common sites of bone metastases include the vertebrae, pelvis, femur and skull and the most frequent symptom is pain, even though 25 percent of patients with bone metastases have no symptoms. Pain may result from direct tumour involvement of bone, with activation of local nociceptors or compression of adjacent nerves, vascular structure and soft tissue. Pain is described as dull and aching and is usually localised to the area of the metastases and is increased by movement. Individual symptoms may vary: for example spine metastases may impinge upon nerve roots and cause radicular pain, whereas patients with metastases to the base of the skull may complain of headaches, or pain in the face, neck or shoulder.

In addition to pain and immobility, complications of bone metastases include:

– pathological fractures, usually in the proximal femur or humerus, most commonly in cancers of the breast, lung, thyroid and in multiple myeloma;
– hypercalcemia, most often observed in cancers of the lung, breast, kidneys and in multiple myeloma; and
– spinal cord compression.

4. *Epidural metastasis/spinal cord compression*

Epidural metastasis is the most threatening complication of bone metastases to the vertebral spine, and becomes truly a medical emergency. Failure to diagnose and treat this condition will lead to permanent neurological deficits. Epidural metastasis is a common complication in patients with breast, prostate or lung cancer, multiple myeloma, renal cell carcinoma or melanoma. The tumour enters the epidural space by continuous spread from adjacent vertebral metastases or from direct invasion of retroperitoneal tumour or tumour located in the posterior thorax through adjacent intervertebral foramina or, rarely from bloodborne seeding of the epidural space. The pain is usually midline although it can also have a radicular distribution, and has a mean duration of 7 weeks prior to the onset of neurological deficits, including motor, sensory and autonomic dysfunctions. More than 70% of these patients with spinal cord compression have an abnormal plain radiograph in the region of pain. In view of the fact that pain is such a reliable early sign, patients should undergo evaluation with magnetic resonance imaging before neurological deficits develop. If MRI is not available, myelograms can be performed. The use of analgesics and corticosteroids are the mainstay of the pharmacological therapy; radiation therapy and surgery or surgery then radiation therapy are standard treatments.

5. *Metastases to the skull*

Middle fossa syndrome. Similar to trigeminal neuralgia, i.e. numbness, paraesthesia, and pain referred to the second or third divisions of the fifth nerve; there could be corresponding sensory deficits and masseter weakness, diplopia, dysarthria, headache and dysphagia related to other cranial nerve damage.

Jugular foramen syndrome. Pain often radiates to the ipsilateral shoulder or neck; may be accompanied by local tenderness and exacerbation with movement of the head. Dysfunction of cranial nerves IX to XII and Horner's syndrome may be present, as well as glossopharyngeal neuralgia.

Clivus metastases. Vertex headache exacerbated by neck flexion with or without neurological dysfuntion.

Orbital & parasellar metastases. Retroorbital or frontal headache, diplopia, visual loss, proptosis and extraocular nerve palsies.

Sphenoid sinus metastases. Bifrontal headache, radiating to both temples with intermittent retro-orbital pain; diplopia and cranial nerve VI palsy.

Occipital condyle invasion. Severe occipital pain, exacerbated by movement with probable XII cranial nerve dysfunction.

Odontoid fracture. Risk of spinal cord compression or transection due to vertebral instability.

6. *Mucositis*

All patients receiving cytotoxic chemotherapy or radiation to the head and neck and to the mediastinum are prone to mucositis. Pain is often severe and interferes with oral intake. Chemotherapy-induced mucositis usually begins 3 to 5 days after therapy is started and reaches its peak at 7 to 10 days, after which it slowly resolves. Clinical signs of mucositis include diminished mucosal thickness and keratinization, superficial sloughing and ulceration. Radiation of the oropharynx and oesophagus results in mucositis, which appears usually at the end of the second week of treatment and tends to disappear around the fourth week; it is sometimes slow in healing and may persist for 2 to 3 weeks after the end of treatment. The mucosa, which initially appears reddened, can be covered with a fibrous exudate as treatment continues.

In both treatments, mucositis pain intensity is related to the extent of tissue damage; pain is described as a burning sensation often accompanied by erythema. Management consists in the use of local analgesics and specific antimicrobial agents.

7. Peripheral neuropathies

Peripheral nerves can be compressed by the tumour or by treatments such as: fibrosis due to radiation treatment, neurotoxic chemotherapy, cutaneous incisions causing the retraction of tissues. Myeloma may cause a progressive painful neuropathy and precedes the onset of other symptoms. This sensorimotor neuropathy is characterised by distal paraesthesias, hypoaesthesia, hyposthenia and muscle wasting and it may occasionally ascend in a manner similar to Guillain–Barré syndrome.

Vincristine, cisplatin and taxol produce dose-related peripheral neuropathies, usually manifested as dysaesthesia in the feet and later in the hands; continuous burning pain is rarely a problem. Vincristine neuropathy may also give rise to cranial neuralgias. The treatment consists in cessation of therapy and administration of analgesics and/or anti-depressants.

8. Plexopathies

Cervical, brachial and lumbosacral plexi can be the origin of unmanageable pain in cancer patients when these structures are infiltrated by tumour or damaged by radiotherapy or compressed by fibrosis after radiotherapy to adjacent structures or if a traction injury related to the positioning of a patient during a prolonged operation exists.

Cervical plexopathy. Pain originating in the cervical plexus radiates into the neck and occiput. It is most commonly caused by metastases to the cervical lymphnodes or the local extension of primary head and neck tumours.

Brachial plexopathy. This is a common complication of breast and lung cancer and lymphoma; it can also be caused by metastasis in the plexus itself from a remote primary tumour. Pain occurs in 85% of patients with brachial plexus involvement and may be present for months before weakness or sensory loss sets in. When the upper plexus is damaged, pain usually begins in the shoulder and is associated with shooting or electrical sensations in the thumb and index finger. When the lower plexus is involved, as is more common, pain begins in the shoulder and radiates into the elbow, arm and into the fourth and fifth digits. Lymphoma may produce brachial plexopathy and spinal cord compression in the absence of vertebral body erosion.

Lumbosacral plexopathy. The lumbosacral plexus may be invaded by tumours of the abdomen and pelvis (colorectal, cervix, endometrial and renal cancers as well as sarcomas and lymphomas); however lumbosacral plexopathies may also be partly metastatic. Pain is usually felt in the lower abdomen, buttock and leg; infiltration of the sacral plexus may produce perineal and perirectal pain. In this plexopathy also, pain precedes the neurological signs of weakness, sensory loss or urinary incontinence by weeks or months. In all cases, an epidural extension of the tumour may occur and in all clinical cases observed, pain precedes the appearance of neurological signs; this calls for prompt recognition of the syndromes and the institution of an adequate treatment can avoid paralysis and incontinence.

Assessment of new pain

Correct pain assessment is an ongoing process requiring constant attention to pain intensity, new pain and to changes in pain patterns, such as a new kind of pain. These may signal new factors such as a fracture, infection or advancement of the disease.

Principles of treatment

It is necessary first of all to distinguish acute pain from chronic pain. The management of acute pain in patients with cancer is similar to the management of patients without cancer; treatment of chronic pain due to cancer requires a different approach. As previously mentioned, a thorough clinical assessment is necessary to determine the type of pain (severity, type, cause,etc.) for appropriate therapeutic modalities. The pathophysiological notion of nociceptive neuropathic and psychogenic pain is of great significance because it leads to the concept of the analgesic ladder which is of great help and very well-known to the majority of doctors and nurses. For good pain control, effective communication is essential, above all to obtain the patient's cooperation.

A multidisciplinary approach is necessary, as well as consideration of all aspects of the patient's suffering. The patient himself should have a clear picture of the planned therapy, as unexpected or sudden changes may otherwise cause him anxiety. Continuity of care is similarly important and repeated assessment is necessary to monitor both pain relief efficacy and side effects of therapy.

Incident pain occurs only in particular circumstances, such as pain that occurs after a particular movement or on standing; this should be treated with local measures including radiotherapy, as well as physical therapy. Analgesics may be used if the pain is mild but if it is severe, it is sometimes preferable to change the patient's activity.

Principles of analgesic use

The choice of which drug to use depends upon the type and severity of the pain, since different analgesics offer different responses. It is important that pain be brought under control as quickly as possible. When prescribing for patients with chronic pain it is commonplace to use a combination of one analgesic drug together with coanalgesic and ajduvant drugs. The use of placebo medications in the treatment of chronic pain due to cancer is not allowed.

The selected drug is prescribed in a dose adequate to manage the pain: the most common failing in the treatment is to give the appropriate drug but in inadequate doses. The scheduling of drugs is according to pharmacokinetics and duration of clinical action. The drug should be given according to a strict schedule in order to prevent the recurrence of pain.

Patients must be informed of potential side effects of treatment, and adequate measures must be taken to prevent them (an example of this is a laxative for constipation due to opioids). The analgesic programme should be as simple as possible, giving preference to mono analgesic drug treatment in oral medication. Continued reassessment of the patient is of great importance in order to individualise patient therapy.

> **The WHO three-step analgesic ladder has been accepted and is used worldwide.**

Non-opioid analgesics

The non-opioid analgesics include salicylates, paracetamol and a series of drugs better known as the non-steroidal anti-inflammatory drugs.

Aspirin

Aspirin is the most frequently used salicylate and the first to be used in clinical treatment.

Characteristics

Absorption & metabolism	Aspirin is rapidly absorbed from the stomach and upper small intestine; it is also hydrolysed by esterases in the plasma, liver and other tissues to the active metabolite, salicylic acid whose plasma half-life is about 2 to 3 hours. Salicylic acid is degraded in the liver and excreted in the urine; excretion is improved by urine alkalinisation.
Action	Aspirin has anti-inflammatory, analgesic and antipyretic effects: the first two relate to a reduced production of prostaglandins in the nearby tissues, due to the inhibition of the cyclo-oxygenase. It is believed that this antipyretic effect acts on the central nervous system.
Dose	The standard dose of aspirin is 10–15 mg/kg. The duration of action is 3 to 4 hours; an average adult of about 60 kg should be given 600–900 mg every 4 hours. An increased dose does not offer better analgesia and may increase the risk of side-effects.
Indications	Aspirin is effective in the management of mild to moderate soft tissue pain and in moderate or severe bone-pain.

Contraindications

Treatment with lower doses is indicated for debilitated cachectic patients as well as for patients with hypoproteinemia, severe hepatic or renal dysfunction; it is contraindicated in patients with a case history of hypersensitivity to aspirin and other NSAIDs. Caution should be taken in patients with thrombocytopenia, coagulation problems and gastritis or ulcer.

Side effects

Gastrointestinal. At least 20% of patients regularly taking aspirin suffer from gastrointestinal toxicity and more may suffer from gastrointestinal blood loss. Aspirin has damaging effects on the mucosa, causing irritation, erosion and ulceration which sometimes causes serious anaemia. The oesophagus and duodenum may be involved. Aspirin produces gastric toxicity by both direct local irritation and by inhibition of prostaglandin synthesis, which leads to secretion of more acid in the stomach and less cytoprotective mucus in the intestine: these latter effects occur if rectal or systemic administration are chosen. The risk of gastrointestinal blood loss increases in persons with peptic ulcer. All patients regularly taking aspirin should be considered candidates for treatment to avoid gastrointestinal complications. Antacids will reduce symptoms but not bleeding; sucralfate or H2-receptor antagonists may reduce the incidence of duodenal ulceration. Misoprostol and omeprazole may be more effective in preventing gastrointestinal toxicity, including gastric erosion and ulceration.

Haemostasis. Aspirin causes loss of platelet aggregation by irreversible inhibition of cyclo-oxygenase in platelets. Prolonged clinical bleeding lasts for 4 to 7 days, until a significant number of platelets appear in the circulation. Aspirin is tightly bound to plasma protein and will displace oral anticoagulants, predisposing to clinical bleeding.

Hypersensitivity reactions. Aspirin may produce a hypersensitivity or allergic reaction in a small but significant proportion of patients. Reactions may occur within minutes of ingestion of small doses of aspirin and may be severe . Patients at risk include those with a history of sensitivity to aspirin or other NSAIDs, patients with asthma, nasal polyposis or an atopic predisposition; aspirin occasionally causes allergies in non-atopic patients. Hypersensitivity reactions include rhinorrhoea, bronchospasm, pruritus, urticaria, angioneurotic oedema and, in more severe cases, laryngeal oedema, anaphylaxis and circulatory collapse. It is important to emphasise that these patients may react similarly to any of the NSAIDs, which therefore should not be prescribed for patients who have demonstrated intolerance to aspirin.

Renal and hepatic dysfunction. Regular ingestion of aspirin may lead to fluid retention and elevation of hepatic enzyme levels but neither are of much clinical significance.

Intoxication. Mild aspirin intoxication causes headache, tinnitus, high frequency deafness, dizziness and nausea. If the treatment is continued it may lead to confusion, drowsiness, hyperventilation and vomiting. These symptoms are caused by free drug concentration in the plasma and are more likely to occur in patients who have a low albumin level or significant liver dysfunction and in individuals taking medication causing urinary acidification, such as ascorbic acid.

Drug interaction. By competitive binding to plasma proteins, aspirin may potentiate the action of oral hypoglycaemic agents.

Available preparations. Aspirin is available in a number of different preparations, most of which are designed to reduce its gastrointestinal toxicity.

- Standard tablets. These are the cheapest form of aspirin but cause the highest incidence of gastrointestinal symptoms and bleeding.
- Soluble Aspirin. These aspirin tablets contain calcium carbonate and citric acid; with this method, dispersion is rapid and there is less gastrointestinal toxicity.
- Buffered Aspirin. These tablets contain antacids or buffers such as magnesium carbonate, aluminium glycinate and magnesium-aluminium hydroxide. The amount of antacid contained in these tablets is too low to alter gastric pH significantly, although the incidence of side-effects may be less than for soluble aspirin.
- Soluble buffered Aspirin. These preparations combine the benefits of the two previous preparations. As-

pro Clear contains 606 mg of sodium bicarbonate in addition to 300 mg of aspirin, significantly lowering the incidence of gastrointestinal toxicity. Alka-Seltzer contains 1.9 g sodium bicarbonate and 324 mg of aspirin: it provides a good absorption of aspirin and also lowers gastrointestinal toxicity; its regular use however, should be limited because of the amount of bicarbonate that would be systemically absorbed.

- Aluminium Aspirin. This type of preparation releases the aspirin mainly in the small intestine and not in the stomach, this reduces gastrointestinal toxicity.
- Glycerine Aspirin. This is highly soluble and is rapidly absorbed in the stomach; it is associated with a low incidence of symptoms or bleeding.
- Enteric-coated Aspirin. This preparation releases aspirin mainly in the small intestine; here also absorption is low and there is a very low incidence of gastric irritation or bleeding.
- Slow-release Aspirin. Microencapsulated aspirin is released slowly in the small intestine and stomach with a very low incidence of gastrointestinal symptoms.
- Rectal and parenteral administration. Absorption of aspirin via rectal administration is slower and less predictable than via the stomach. This may cause gastric irritation and bleeding by inhibition of gastric prostaglandin synthesis.

The best administration for continued use of aspirin is the soluble type.

Table 1.

Analgesic	T1\2	ORAL DOSE (max.mg/day)	DT (hours)	Side Effects
Aspirin	3–5	500–1000, (4000)	4–6	GI toxicity +++, bleeding +++, PLT ++
Diclofenac	3	50	6–8	Dispepsia+++, Bleeding ++
Diflunisal	8–12	500–1000, (1500)	8–12	Dispepsia+
Droxicam	45	20	24	Dispepsia ++, Bleeding ++
Flurbiprofen	3.5	300	8	Dispepsia++
Ibuprofen	2–4	200–400, (2400)	4–6	Dispepsia+, Bleeding +
Indomethacin	4–5	50–100, (200)	8–12, 24	Dispepsia+++, Bleeding +++, Confusion +++, Depression +++
Ketoprofen	1.5	50–100, (300)	4–8	Dispepsia+
Ketorolac	5	10–20, (60)	6–8	Dispepsia++, Bleeding, ++, Confusion +
Mefenamic Acid	3, 5	1000	6	Dispepsia ++
Methamizol	6, 9	500–1000	4–6	Dispepsia++
Naproxen	13	250–500, (1250)	6–8	Dispepsia+, Bleeding +
Na-Naproxen	13	275–500, (1375)	6–8	Dispepsia+, Bleeding ++
Piroxicam	45	20, (40)	24	Dispepsia++, Bleeding ++

Other salicylates

Other salicylates include cation salicylates, magnesium trisalicylate and diflunisal.

Diflunisal. This is a difluorophenyl preparation, a synthetic derivative of salicylic acid. It is well absorbed after oral administration and causes less gastric irritation. It has a plasma half-life of 8 to 12 hours and can be given twice daily. Diflunisal is not converted to salicylic acid and its exact mechanism of action is unknown. Similar to aspirin it inhibits prostaglandin production and at high doses it inhibits platelet aggregation. It is an effective analgesic in conditions like osteoarthritis and on pain from skeletal and soft tissue metastases. It has little antipyretic activity and the recommended dosage is 500 mg two to four times a day.

Cation salicylates are best avoided in view of their high side effects as well as their high cost whereas magnesium salicylate is soluble, well absorbed with a longer plasma half-life and well-tolerated.

Paracetamol

Paracetamol and phenacetin, synthetic derivatives of acetanilid have analgesic and antipyretic properties.

Absorption and metabolism. Paracetamol is rapidly absorbed mainly from the small intestine. It has a plasma half-life of about 2 hours. The drug is conjugated in the liver and excreted in the urine. If high doses are administered, the hepatic system may become saturated: this can cause hepatic necrosis.

Action. Paracetamol has analgesic and antipyretic properties similar to aspirin but has no anti-inflammatory action. It appears to act by inhibition of prostaglandin synthesis and has more effect on the central nervous system.

Indications and contraindications. Paracetamol is indicated for mild to moderate bone or soft tissue pain related to cancer. It is the non-opioid drug of choice for patients with hypersensitivity to aspirin or NSAIDs and for all those for whom NSAIDs are contraindicated. Paracetamol should be given with caution to patients with severely compromised liver function.

Dose. It may be administered orally or rectally. The advisable dose for adults is 500–1000 mg every 4 to 6 hours.

Side effects. Unlike aspirin, paracetamol does not cause gastric irritation and does not interfere with platelet function. At normal therapeutic dose it is well tolerated. It is rare that patients develop constipation or allergic rash. Chronic ingestion of 4–6 g per day may cause

hepatotoxicity with mild elevation of hepatic enzyme levels which is reversible in any case. There may be a slight prolongation of the prothrombin ratio which may necessitate adjustment of any anticoagulant treatment.

Non-steroidal anti-inflammatory drugs

Action, pharmacology. The NSAIDs have anti-inflammatory, analgesic and anti-pyretic effects. There is considerable variability in the pharmacokinetic properties of the various drugs which results in a variation of frequency of administration. They are all well absorbed by the oral route and some are effective when administered rectally. The mechanism of action is by inhibition of prostaglandin synthesis even though some side effects may be mediated via the central nervous system.

Indications and contraindications. These are indicated for the treatment of moderate cancer-related pain in bone and soft tissue. They are contraindicated for patients with documented hypersensitivity to aspirin or other NSAIDs. Relative contraindications include the presence of peptic ulceration, thrombocytopenia, bleeding diathesis and severe hepatic or renal dysfunction.

Side effects. Very similar to aspirin.

Gastrointestinal. The most frequent side effect is gastrointestinal irritation with erosion, ulceration and bleeding. Studies in patients with rheumatic disorders suggest the frequency of gastrointestinal toxicity is less than with aspirin. Chronic use of NSAIDs often causes constipation, exceptions being indomethacin and flurbiprofen, which, on the contrary may cause diarrhoea.

Haemostasis. NSAIDs cause platelet dysfunction by inhibition of platelet prostaglandin synthetase; the inhibition however, unlike with aspirin is reversible once the drug is discontinued and the bleeding tendency resolves within a few days.

Central nervous system. The side effects include headache, drowsiness, dizziness, euphoria and occasionally psychoses.

Renal. NSAIDs may cause sodium and fluid retention. This dysfunction is all the more serious in patients with previous renal impairment and the treatment may inhibit the action of frusemide and other cardiovascular drugs. It may also cause interstitial nephritis and papillary necrosis but this occurs infrequently and usually only after prolonged use.

Others. Cases of hypersensitivity or allergic reactions have been reported as well as skin rashes and reversible increase of hepatic enzymes; the latter is rarely of clinical significance but the drugs should still be given with caution to patients with severe hepatic dysfunction; rare cases of agranulocytosis have been reported.

NSAIDS for patients with cancer

The reason for the use of NSAIDs in cancer patients is that their analgesic and anti-inflammatory effect is at least equivalent to aspirin with less gastrointestinal toxicity and with fewer tablets to be taken.

Ibuprofen has a good anti-inflammatory action with significantly fewer side effects than indomethacin. The dose is 400 mg orally, 6-8 hourly.

Flurbiprofen, 100mg every 8 hours, seems to be just as effective as the latter and is less toxic.

Naproxen causes gastrointestinal and CNS side effects with about the same frequency as indomethacin. The usual dose is 250–750 mg orally every 12 hours or 500mg by suppositories.

Indomethacin, introduced in the 1960's, is a potent prostaglandin synthetase inhibitor and has a significant analgesic and anti-inflammatory action. However, in view of the high incidence of its side effects it is not often used. Of all NSAIDs, it has the highest rate of gastrointestinal toxicity and a significant number of patients particularly the elderly, develop neurological side effects. Fluid retention, neutropenia and thrombocytopenia may occur, although they are usually reversible if the treatment is withdrawn. Aplastic anaemia is rare. The usual dose is 25mg orally every 6 hours or 100mg by suppositories, the latter having significant local side effects when they are used on a chronic basis.

Opioid analgesics

Mechanism of action
The opioid analgesics exert their effect by interaction with the opioid receptors in the brain and the spinal cord. There are a number of different types of opioid receptors, the main ones being mu, delta and kappa, which normally interact with a range of endogenous opioid substances including, endorphins and enkephalins. The effective role of these substances and the different effects

of activation of the various receptors are still not fully understood.

Classification
The opioid analgesics are classified as natural opium alkaloids, semi-synthetic or synthetic, and as agonist or antagonist on the basis of their receptor interactions.

- An agonist drug is one that binds to a particular receptor and produces a physiological effect (for example analgesia obtained by means of mu receptor stimulation);
- An antagonist drug is one that binds to a receptor but does not produce any physiological effect and may interfere with the binding of the agonist to or displace it from the receptor (naloxone);
- A mixed agonist-antagonist is a drug that has agonist effects when given alone but that may act as an antagonist if administered with an agonist. There are those that are antagonists only at higher doses (e.g. buprenorphine) and those that are antagonists at any dose (e.g. pentazocine). Buprenorphine, if given alone, has an agonist effect; given in low doses with another agonist it will have no detrimental effect but if given in higher doses with another agonist it will have antagonist action and may increase pain and withdrawal symptoms. Similarly, pentazocine if given alone has an agonist action but given in any dose with another agonist it will have antagonist action and may precipitate pain and withdrawal symptoms.
- Opioids are the major class of analgesics used in the management of moderate to severe pain, because of their effectiveness, ease of titration and favourable risk-to-benefit ratio. Opioids produce analgesia by binding to specific receptors both within and outside the CNS.

The most commonly used full agonists include morphine, hydromorphone, codeine, oxycodone, hydrocodone, methadone, levorphanol and fentanyl. These opioids are classified as full agonists because they do not have a ceiling to their analgesic effect and will not antagonise the effects of other agonists. Side effects include constipation, nausea, urinary retention, confusion, sedation and respiratory depression.

- Buprenorphine is a partial agonist. It has a relatively low intrinsic efficacy at the opioid receptor.

Mixed agonist-antagonists block opioid analgesia at one type of opioid receptor (mu or kappa). Patients being treated with opioid agonists should not be given mixed agonist-antagonist, because this may cause withdrawal symptoms.

Morphine is the most commonly used opioid because of its availability in a wide variety of dosage forms. Its pharmacokinetic and pharmacodynamic preparations are known and is relatively cheap.

Meperidine may be used for short periods to treat acute pain and to manage rigours induced by medication, but it should be avoided in cancer patients because of its short duration of action and its toxic metabolite, normeperidine. This metabolite accumulates, particularly when renal function is impaired and causes CNS stimulation, which may in turn cause dysphoria, agitation and convulsions.

Morphine myths are still an obstacle in daily practice.

1. Tolerance and physical dependence

Opioid tolerance and physical dependence are expected with long-term opioid treatment and should not be confused with psychological dependence, manifested as drug abuse behaviour.

Physical dependence on opioids is revealed when the drug is abruptly discontinued or when naloxone is administered, and is typically manifested as anxiety, irritability, chills and even hot flushes, joint pain, lacrimation, rhinorrhoea, diaphoresis, nausea, vomiting, abdominal cramps and diarrhoea. In the milder forms of the opioid abstinence syndrome it is mistaken for a viral "flu-like' syndrome. For opioids with short half-lives (i.e., codeine, hydrocodone, morphine, hydromorphone), the onset of withdrawal symptoms can occur within 6–12 hours and peak at 24–72 hours after drug discontinuation. For opioids with long half-lives (methadone, levorphanol, transdermal fentanyl) the onset of withdrawal may be delayed for 24 hours or more after drug discontinuation and may be of milder intensity.

Patients with cancer occasionally require withdrawal of the treatment or rapid decrease of the dose when the cause of the pain is effectively eliminated by anti neoplastic treatments or pain perception is modified by neurolytic or neurosurgical procedures. In such cases, the opioid abstinence syndrome can be avoided by gradual withdrawal of the drug. For morphine treatment:

– reduce by 50% the initial dose, the first 2 days;

– reduce by 25% the daily dose over a five-day period.

Transdermal clonidine (0.1 to 0.2 mg/day) can be administered subcutaneously to reduce anxiety, tachycardia and other autonomic symptoms that are associated with opioid withdrawal.

Tolerance to opioids is defined as a necessity to increase dose requirements to obtain the same effect. For many cancer patients, the first sign of tolerance is a decrease in the duration of analgesia for a given dose; increasing dose requirements are most consistently correlated with progression of the disease, which causes pain intensity.

Patients with stable disease rarely require increased doses.

2. Dosage titration

Opioid doses should be adjusted to attain pain relief with an acceptable level of adverse effects. Dosages should be frequently adjusted. There is no ceiling or maximal recommended dose, and in fact, very large doses may be required for very severe pain. The dose that is required is the dose that is effective. Occasionally, the number of pills (or the number of patches e.g. fentanyl) may limit the amount of drug by the route.

Effective pain relief is obtained by the anticipation and prevention of pain. Because many patients have persistent pain, it is important to use opioids at regular intervals rather than only when needed. This use of 'as needed' dosing should be allowed only during the first 24–48 hours, when a new drug is started in order to define the best adequate dose for that individual patient.

Table 2. Opioid analgesics

	Parenteral		Oral	
morphine	10 mg	q 3–4 h	30 mg	q 3–4 h
morphine controlled release			90–120 mg	q 12 h
buprenorphine	0.3 mg	6–8 h	0.4 mg sl	6–8 h
codeine	120 mg	—	200 mg	—
diamorphine (heroin)	4 mg	3–4 h	20 mg	3–4 h
hydromorphone	1.5 mg	q 3–4 h	7.5 mg	q 3–4 h
levorphanol	2 mg	q 6–8 h	4 mg	q 6–8 h
methadone	10 mg	q 6–8 h	20 mg	q 6–8 h
oxycodone	—	—	30 mg	q 3–4 h
meperidine	100 mg	q 3 h	200 mg	q 2–3 h

Note: Transdermal fentanyl is an alternative option. Transdermal fentanyl dosage is not calculated as equianalgesic tp a single morphine dose. Doses above 25 ug/h should not be used in opioid-naive patients.

Pain management of moderate to severe pain should be with oral opioids in combination with an NSAID or paracetamol. The optimal dose will control pain with few side effects such as sedation, constipation or nausea.

Adjuvant drugs may be used to counteract the predictable side effects of opioids: for example dietary caffeine supplementation to counteract opioid-induced sedation, antiemetic drugs for opioid-induced nausea, laxatives to counteract constipation etc.

It is usually advisable to observe the patient's response to several different opioids before routes of administration are changed or an anaesthetic, neurosurgical or other invasive approach to relieve persistent pain is attempted. For example, patients who continue to experience nausea, sedation or mental clouding on oral morphine should be switched to an equianalgesic dose of an other opioid such as hydromorphone, fentanyl, methadone.

All analgesics, except morphine, have a maximal dose per day limit.

Morphine does not have a maximal dose per day limit and the dose can be increased (without limits) providing continuous pain-relief.

3. Routes of administration

The onset of analgesic effect and duration of action for an opioid depends on the specific drug chosen and its formulation. Most are well absorbed after oral or rectal administration, even though absorption may not be complete. Drugs absorbed from the gut are subject to first-pass metabolism in the liver and should therefore be given orally rather than parenterally.

Oral: The oral route is the preferred route because it is the most convenient. Oral opioids are available in tablets, capsule and liquid forms, and in immediate and controlled-release formulations. Controlled-release tablets become immediately released when crushed and therefore are not appropriate for patients who are unable to swallow whole tablets. A certain percentage of patients may require alternative routes during their illness, for example should complications arise such as mucositis or in the terminal phase. Therefore, when patients cannot take medications orally, other less invasive routes such as rectal or transdermal routes should be tried; subcutaneous infusion may be eventually used.

Transdermal: The transdermal route for opioid delivery provides a simple and convenient method for administering the strong opioid, fentanyl on a continuous basis. This route obviates the need for parenteral administration, and most importantly, provides a unique approach for the patient who cannot or will not take oral drugs. Studies to date on the clinical usefulness of this route compared to other approaches demonstrate its efficacy and safety. Some recent studies suggest that compared to oral morphine, transdermal fentanyl may be associated with less nausea, vomiting and constipation. The dose conversion from oral morphine (100 mg/24 hrs) to TTS-fentanyl is a 25 ug/hr patch. This is the starting dose with dose adjustment based on the patient's degree of pain relief and side effects. Following application of the patch, analgesia is maintained for 72 hours. Rarely, patients may require replacement at 48 hours. When starting a patient on a patch, analgesic medication should be made available to the patient during the initial titration phase with rescue medications available to the patient for breakthrough pain. The availability of an alternative opioid drug to morphine in patch form provides clinicians with a wider range of opioid drugs, facilitating their availability to individualise drug treatment for patients

who are unable to tolerate morphine because of excessive side effects or unable to take opioids by the oral route.

Intravenous or subcutaneous: Both these routes of administration are effective alternatives, the patients, however, who may benefit from continuous infusion of opioids are:

– those with persistent nausea and vomiting;
– those with severe dysphagia or swallowing disorders;
– those with delirium, confusion, stupor or other mental status changes that make oral administration difficult because of risks of aspiration in an unprotected airway;
– those who require high doses necessitating numerous tablets;
– those who experience side effects in relation to each dose of an "as-needed medication;
– those who require rapid incremental doses of analgesia.

Among the main benefits of opioid infusions, compared with intermittent administration, is the lower quantity of injections required. The intravenous route provides the most rapid onset of analgesia, but the duration of analgesia after a bolus dose is shorter than with other routes.

A continuous intravenous infusion provides the most consistent level of analgesia and is easily accomplished for patients who have permanent intravenous access for other purposes. If intravenous access is not desirable, continuous subcutaneous opioid infusion is a valid alternative, which apart from being practical also at home, provides levels in blood comparable to those with intravenous doses. Initial doses are the same as those for intravenous administration, however during intravenous treatment the dose needs to be increased rapidly in view of the rapid drug tolerance.

> Intramuscular administration of drugs should be avoided because this route is painful and absorption is not reliable.

Rectal: The rectal route may be used when patients have nausea or vomiting or are in a preoperative or postoperative phase. The rectal route is contraindicated if there are lesions of the anus or rectum because placement of the suppository will cause pain. This route is also to be avoided if there is diarrhoea or in elderly or infirm patients who are physically unable to place the suppository. Suppositories of morphine, hydromorphone and oxymorphone are commercially available.

Patient-Controlled Analgesia (PCA): Patient-Controlled Analgesia allows the patient himself to control the amount of analgesia he receives. This is commonly done by the oral route or by the use of a special drug-delivery pump that can be set to administer the drug intravenously, subcutaneously, epidurally or intraspinally.

Intraspinal: Analgesics may be administered intraspinally when pain cannot be controlled in any other way because side effects such as confusion and nausea limit the possibility of dose escalation. The intraspinal route is to be taken into consideration when maximal doses via other routes fail. This route requires

professional experience, significant family support and sophisticated follow up.

As with systemic opioid administration, the dose range depends on the level of pain and tolerance. Any agent delivered into the epidural or intrathecal space should be pure because additional substances can produce neurotoxicity. Morphine is the most commonly used intraspinal drug; others are hydromorphone, fentanyl or sufentanil and may be useful substitutes for patients suffering from side effects due to morphine. Intraspinal morphine may produce the same side effects as in other routes of administration because epidural or subarachnoid morphine is absorbed into the circulation by way of the epidural vascular plexus. A 10mg dose of morphine produces levels in blood comparable to an intramuscular injection of the same dose. Very lipophilic opioids such as fentanyl and sufentanil have a more limited CSF distribution but can also gain access to the blood.

In some patients, it is possible to give relatively small doses of opioid spinally and produce pain relief while avoiding the side effects that can limit oral or parenteral administration.

The main indication for the long-term administration of intraspinal opioids is intractable pain in the lower part of the body particularly when the pain is bilateral or midline. Opioids (sometimes coadministered with other agents such as local anaesthetic) are delivered to the epidural or subarachnoid space via percutaneously placed catheters; external catheters can be used for short-term treatment whereas for more prolonged treatment, the delivery system must be internalised. Side effects include the development of tolerance, urinary retention, constipation, pruritus, device failure and infection.

Intraventricular: Intraventricular administration produces beneficial effects in recalcitrant pain due to head and neck cancer that affect the brachial plexus. Small doses of morphine (less than 5mg/day) are enough to obtain adequate analgesia. Complications are rare, the most important being infection; tolerance and respiratory depression are negligible. Intraventricular morphine requires the placement of a catheter connected to a subcutaneous reservoir for intermittent administration or an infusion pump for continuous infusion. Although the use of this method is still very limited, experience with intraventricular morphine administration is steadily increasing.

4. Management of side effects

Constipation and sedation are the most common side effects associated with opioids; others include confusion, nausea, vomiting, respiratory depression, dry mouth, urinary retention, pruritus, myoclonus, altered cognitive function, euphoria, sleep disturbances, sexual dysfuntion, physiological dependence, tolerance and inappropriate secretion of antidiuretic hormone. Because there is great individual variation in the development of opioid-induced side effects, they should be monitored carefully for and the most common ones anticipated and treated.

Constipation: constipation is such a common problem in patients treated with opioids that prophylactic treatment with laxatives is compulsory. Tolerance to the constipating effects of opioids eit-

her does not occur or occurs very slowly during chronic therapy. It may worsen with time because of the disease process (e.g. intestinal obstruction, paralytic ileus due to spinal cord compression, decreased food and fluid intake due to anorexia). Mild constipation can be treated by an increase in fibre consumption and the use of laxatives such as milk of magnesia. These should be administered regularly unless there are contraindications. Severe constipation occurs as a result of the inhibition of peristalsis by opioids and can be treated with a stimulating cathartic drug, such as standardised senna concentrate or hyperosmotic agents like lactulose. Emollient laxatives are of limited usefulness because of colonic resorption of water from the forming stool. They should therefore be used in combination with stimulant laxatives to ease defecation, especially in bedridden patients.

Sedation: transitory sedation is common when opioid doses are increased, but tolerance usually sets in rapidly, 2 to 4 days Persistent drug-induced sedation is usually best treated by reduction of the opioid in each dose and increase in the dosage frequency. This strategy will decrease the peak concentrations in blood (and brain) while maintaining the same total dose. In some patients, switching to another opioid may reduce the sedative effects. CNS stimulants such as caffeine, dextroamphetamine (2.5–7.5 mg twice daily, orally), or methylphenidate (5 to 10 mg/day, orally) can be helpful. These agents increase the cognitive function of patients receiving opioids.

Nausea and vomiting: There are no controlled studies that establish the indications, efficacy and dosing requirements for treatment of opioid-induced nausea and vomiting. Clinical experience suggests that these side effects can be managed with antiemetics chosen according to their mode of action. Metoclopramide is helpful when neuroleptics such as prochlorperazine, chlorpromazine or haloperidol fail. Scopolamine, an acetylcholine receptor antagonist, can be given transdermally to reduce nausea due to motion sickness or related to cancer and ameliorate symptoms, as a result of its effect on the vestibular system. When patients complain of nausea and vomiting it is often helpful to administer an antiemetic on a fixed schedule for several days, after which as-needed dosing is usually adequate. Depending on the antiemetic chosen, patients should be monitored for the possibility of increased sedation.

Respiratory depression: Patients receiving long-term opioid therapy usually develop tolerance to the respiratory-depressant effects of these agents. Occasionally, respiratory depression occurs when pain is abruptly relieved and the sedative effects of opioids are no longer opposed by the stimulating effects of pain. In a symptomatic patient, physical stimulation may be enough to prevent significant hypoventilation. Opioid antagonists like naloxone should be given cautiously to patients who are being treated with opioids on a long-term basis. Because patients who have become tolerant to opioids show great sensitivity to the effects of antagonist drugs, symptomatic respiratory depression should be treated carefully with a dilute solution of naloxone (0.4 mg in 10 ml of saline), administered as 0.5 ml (0.02 mg) boluses every minute. The dose of naloxone should be titrated to the patient's respiratory rate. Naloxone should be given in doses that improve respiratory function but do not reverse analgesia.

Far more common than acute respiratory depression is subacute overdose, in which sedation gradually builds and is followed by a slowing respiratory rate and then by ventilatory failure. The degree of sedation rather than the respiratory rate is a better indicator of impending respiratory depression. The risk of this complication is highest during titration of opioids with long plasma half-lives such as methadone and levorphanol.

Clinicians are often concerned that high doses of opioids may harm or even kill a patient, particularly when doses are further increased to alleviate pain. This double effect is seen with any medication, the administration of which is always a risk-versus-benefit calculation; taking into consideration that if the patient's death is imminent, the benefit of painless death is preferable to the increased risk of earlier death.

> Because many patients in the terminal phase have been receiving opioid pain medications over a significant period, the fear of shortening life by medication is usually unfounded, in fact tolerance sets in without respiratory compromise.

Other side effects: Opioids occasionally cause myoclonus, seizures, hallucinations, confusion, sexual dysfunction, sleep disturbance and pruritus. Prolonged used is known to affect libido in both men and women. Women experience amenorrhoea and infertility whereas men report an inability to maintain erection. Changes in serum testosterone have been described and may be responsible for some of these effects. Urinary retention may also occur, especially with spinal opioids in men with prostatism or in patients with pelvic tumours and bladder outlet obstruction. Management of these side effects may include discontinuation of adjuvant drugs with potentiating effects (e.g. tricyclic antidepressants) or changing of the type of analgesic or route of administration. Diphenhydramine, an antihistamine, may reduce pruritus in some patients. The syndrome of the inappropriate secretion of antidiuretic hormone is a rare, often transitory, adverse effect of opioid drugs, most commonly reported with morphine and methadone.

Adjuvant analgesics

The adjuvant analgesics and co-analgesic drugs, whilst not true analgesics in the pharmacological sense, may contribute substantially to pain relief when used either alone or in combination with other analgesics. They may have an analgesic-sparing effect and should be considered in the treatment of all types of pain related to advanced cancer. They are of particular clinical importance in the treatment of pain relatively unresponsive to morphine, including neuropathic pain and that due to raised intracranial pressure. Adjuvant analgesics are: corticosteroids, progestogens, anticonvulsants, antidepressants, neuroleptics, anxiolytics, psychostimulants, oral local anaesthetic agents and antibiotics.

Corticosteroids: Corticosteroids are effective co-analgesics in many situations. They act by inhibition of prostaglandin production with reduction of inflammation and oedema associated with tumour deposits. For patients with lymphoproliferative disorders and a few with breast cancer, they also offer an antitumour action. Corticosteroids are particularly useful in the treatment of neurological disturbances secondary to metastatic cancer. The pain related to intracranial pressure and extradural spinal cord compression are usually promptly relieved. The same may be said of pain associated with tumour compression or invasion of the brachial or lumbosacral plexus or other nerve roots. When neurological function is compromised, the use of corticosteroids may prevent further deterioration.

They are also effective in treating the pain of bone metastases and that due to capsular stretching by metastases in the liver and other viscera. They may be of benefit in pain associated with soft tissue infiltration, especially in the head and neck, abdomen and pelvis. Pain associated with vena cava superior obstruction and lymphoedema may also be reduced. The generalised bone and endosteal pain associated with haematological malignancies, as well as the pain related to hepatosplenomegaly or lymphadenopathy, frequently respond to corticosteroids. They are of less common use as adjuvant analgesics to treat the pain of metastases to joints and tenesmus associated with rectal tumours.

The commonly used corticosteroids are prednisolone, dexamethasone and hydrocortisone. Approximate equivalent doses are 30mg of prednisolone, 4mg of dexamethasone and 120mg of hydrocortisone. These doses refer to the anti-inflammatory and glucocorticoid effects of the drugs. There is also a variation between the mineralcorticoid effect of the drugs, which leads to salt and water retention and oedema. Hydrocortisone has a higher mineralcorticoid effect than prednisolone, which in turn has more than dexamethasone.

In practice, dexamethasone or methylprednisolone are the drugs usually used for the treatment of pain caused by raised intracranial pressure and spinal cord compression. For other indications, prednisolone 15–30mg/d is frequently effective; treatment may be ini-

Table 3. Adjuvant drugs

Drug	Dose (mg die) oral route	Indications
CORTICOSTEROIDS		
methylprednisoline	125 e.v.	
prednisone	5–15	
	50	perineural edema, anorexia
dexamethasone	4–12	neural compression, increased
	16–24 e.v.	intracranial pressure and spinal cord
	80–100	compression
NEUROLEPTICS		
chlorpromazine	10–25	
haloperidol	2.5–5	
prochlorperazine	5–10	vomiting
BISPHOSPHONATES		
etidronate	7.5 mg/kg IV	
pamidronate	30–60 mg IV	hypercalcaemia and bone pain metastases
ANTIDEPRESSANTS		
amitriptyline	25–100	
chlorimipramine	25–100	
trazodone	150	dysesthetic, postherpetic
fluvoxamine	100–300	neuralgia and depression
fluoxetine	20	
ANTICONVULSANTS		
carbamazepine	400–600	
sodium valproate	400–600	neural compression, neural infiltration
phenytoine	300	and neuropathic pain
clonazepam	0,5–1 kg	
BENZODIAZEPINES		
alprazolam	0.25–0.50	anxiety, contractures and insomnia
diazepam	10	
triazolam	0,25	
oxazepam	20	
LOCAL ANAESTHETICS		
mexiletine	10/kg	diabetic neuropathy, trigeminal
tocainide	20/kg	neuralgia and neuropathic pain
	5/kg iv/s	

tiated however at a higher dose, after which it may be gradually reduced.

The effects of corticosteroids are usually seen within a few hours or a few days of initial treatment.

The side effects of corticosteroids are related to both the dose employed and the duration of treatment. For patients with advanced cancer, the clinical importance of these side effect depends very much on the patient's anticipated life expectancy.

Gastrointestinal side effects occur relatively frequently with corticosteroids. Patients frequently complain of epigastric pain or indigestion, which may be symptomatically treated with antacids. Corticosteroids may aggravate an already existing peptic ulceration or erosions and cause pain and bleeding, particularly when used in combination with aspirin or an NSAID. An H2-receptor antagonist may protect against the development of duodenal ulceration; the prostaglandin analogue, misoprostol, may protect against gastric ulceration.

Other side effects of corticosteroids are of variable clinical importance. The production or aggravation of diabetes may occur. Abrupt withdrawal of steroids may cause hypoadrenalism with weakness, hypotension, hypoglycemia, headache, nausea and vomiting, and restlessness, as well as muscle and joint pain. Stimulation of appetite and some weight gain may be considered beneficial by some patients with disseminated cancer. Fluid retention and oedema are not usually troublesome except with high doses but care must be taken in patients with hypertension and cardiac or renal disease. Patients taking corticosteroids for more than a few weeks will develop a Cushingoid appearance, to some degree, depending on the dose.

There may be subjective improvement in muscle strength, which is often transient. Chronic administration of corticosteroids may lead to proximal myopathy and weakness, which may be debilitating. Some patients develop a syndrome of steroid pseudo-rheumatism with pain in the muscles, tendons and joints, but this is rare. Chronic corticosteroid therapy, as given to some patients with haematological malignancies or cerebral tumours, may lead to osteoporosis and, less frequently, aseptic necrosis of the femoral or humeral head. Corticosteroids predispose to infection, particularly oral candidiasis and acneiform skin lesions; of more importance, they may cover up the signs and symptoms of infection.

The neuropsychological side effects of corticosteroids are variable; there is generally some euphoria and an improved sense of well-being, which may be of benefit in the palliative care setting. Many patients may also develop a certain degree of insomnia which is reduced if the drug is taken before midday following the variation in endogenous cortisol; less frequently, they may develop more serious side effects including agitation, hypomania, depression or even frank psychosis.

Progestogens: Progestational agents, such as medroxyprogesterone acetate and megestrol acetate are used to manage pain related to metastatic disease in patients with breast, prostate, endometrial and renal cancer. Progestogen therapy may have an antitumour action in some patients with these diseases, but the co-analgesic effect occurs in a significantly larger percentage of the patients. The mechanism by which progestogens might exert this effect is unknown. The commonly employed doses are 200–500mg/d of medroxyprogesterone acetate or 160mg/d of megestrol acetate. The side effects of progestogen therapy include nausea and vomiting, fluid retention leading to weight gain, oedema, cardiac failure, hypertension and vaginal bleeding.

Whilst treatment with progestogens may be of benefit in the small proportions of patients who achieve objective tumour response, their role as co-analgesics in other patients remains to be established. The frequency of the side effects, at the recommended doses, precludes their general use for patients with advanced cancer.

Anticonvulsants: Anticonvulsants may be of benefit in the treatment of neuropathic pain resulting from infiltration of the brachial, coeliac or lumbosacral plexus, post-herpetic or post-surgical neuralgia, phantom limb pain and other painful neuropathies.

The anticonvulsants presumably act by suppression of spontaneous neuronal discharges and neuronal hyperexcitability that occur after nerve injury. They may be also more effective against the shooting stabbing components of neuropathic pain and have less effect on the burning dysaesthetic discomfort which frequently occurs.

The anticonvulsants most frequently used in the treatment of this pain include carbamazepine, phenytoin, sodium valproate and clonazepan. The dose is the same as or much higher than the one used for anticonvulsant therapy, although there are no data relating to blood levels and analgesic activity. The dose should be reduced if toxicity ensues. Serum levels can be checked and if there is no response when the levels are in the therapeutic range for anticonvulsant therapy, the drug should be stopped. There is a considerable variation between the drugs, suggesting a lack of cross-resistance and should therapy with one drug fail, treatment with a second anticonvulsant is sometimes successful.

The side effects of the different anticonvulsants are similar, with gastric intolerance (nausea and vomiting), sedation, ataxia, dizziness and confusion. Carbamazepine may also cause leucopenia, therefore the peripheral white blood cell count should be checked periodically. The sedative effects will be additive with those of any antidepressants or opioid analgesics being used, therefore individualisation of the doses may be necessary.

Bisphosphonates: Bone pain is a frequent complication of bone metastases. It is probably caused by osteoclast-induced bone resorption by the tumour, which may also result in osteoporosis, hypercalcemia, microfractures or pathologic fractures. Bisphosphonates (e.g. etidronate, pamidronate) are analogues of endogenous pyrophosphates, which inhibit bone resorption in vivo. They are available for the management of hypercalcemia associated with malignancy. Relief of bone pain or decreased analgesic use after commencement of the drug has been reported.

Calcitonin is also a strong inhibitor of osteoclast-induced bone resorption and is used in the treatment of hypercalcemia due to malignancy.

Antidepressants: Antidepressants may add to analgesia by increasing nighttime sedation and improving mood; these effects may be seen with any of the antidepressants including tricyclic (amitriptyline, clorimipramine imipramine, doxepin), tetracyclic (mianserin), monoamine oxidator inhibitors and other drugs.

The tricyclic antidepressants may also be of use as adjuvant analgesics in the treatment of neuropathic pain. The mechanism of action is thought to relate to blocking the re-uptake of serotonin in the central nervous system. These effects occur with much lower doses than are used for the treatment of depression and may be seen within 24-48 hours of start of treatment. A low dose trial treatment with tricyclic antidepressant is advisable in patients with neuropathic pain that is not easily controlled with other analgesics. For neuropathic pain, amitriptyline is started at a dose of 25mg at night and slowly increased to 50–75mg at night; other tricyclic drugs may be used at equivalent doses. Should one drug fail, another type can give good relief to the patient. The side effects of these lower doses are usually mild.

Neuroleptics:

–   *Phenothiazines.* The phenothiazine tranquillisers, with one exception, have no analgesic action but may be of benefit because they reduce anxiety and improve night-time sedation. However, unless a phenothiazine is indicated for the treatment of delirium or nausea, the same benefits may be obtained with a benzodiazepine without the potentially troublesome anticholinergic side effects of phenothiazines.
    The phenothiazine drug that has been shown to have analgesic properties is methotrimeprazine or levopromazine (Nozinan or Levoprome). It is particularly useful in patients with respiratory depression or bowel obstruction and in whom a reduction of opioid analgesics is preferable; its additional benefits are antiemetic and antianxiety effects. The usual dose is 10–20 mg given every 4–6 hours; an injection of 5mg of methotrimeprazine should be given as a test dose to observe both its sedative and hypotensive effects. Side effects of methotrimeprazine include sedation, postural hypotension and extrapyramidal effects. Because of its sedative and hypotensive effects it is recommended for non-ambulant patients. The strong sedative and hypnotic effects may limit the use of the drug in a patient who is ambulatory.

–   *Butyrophenones.* Haloperidol, like chlorpromazine, will produce sedation and reduce anxiety. Haloperidol however has no intrinsic analgesic activity and equivalent results can be obtained with anxiolytic drugs that do not have the sedative, anticholinergic and hallucinatory side effects of haloperidol.

Anxiolytic drugs:

–   *Benzodiazepines.* In this group we have diazepam, oxazepam and alprazolam, which are frequently used in patients with advanced cancer. They do not have analgesic action but may be of benefit to patients in view of their anxiolytic effect. Diazepam is of particular use in patients with muscle spasm or acute musculoskeletal pain. Side effects include drowsiness, weakness and postural hypotension.

–   *Antihistamines.* Some antihistamines, for example hydroxyzine, do have some analgesic action. Hydroxyzine may have some opioid-sparing action but this is probably due to the sedative anxiolytic action of the drug rather than intrinsic analgesic activity. The dose of hydroxyzine is 10–25mg three times a day. Its main side effect is sedation.

Psychostimulants:

- *Cocaine.* Controlled studies have shown no additional analgesic effect when cocaine is given in addition to morphine or heroin. Administration of cocaine leads to a transient improvement of well being and strength but these effects usually last only a few days. In the elderly or debilitated, cocaine may cause agitation and confusion.
- *Amphetamines.* Amphetamines potentiate the action of opioid analgesics in postoperative patients, but it is uncertain whether or not this effect is maintained in chronic treatment. In patients with advanced cancer, amphetamines will counteract sedation caused by opioid drugs and permit adequate analgesia with tolerable side effects. Tachyphylaxis and dependence may develop quickly, necessitating an increase of the dosage and elderly patients are prone to dysphoric side effects.
- *Methylphenidate.* Methylphenidate has no analgesic action but can be used to counteract sedation caused by opioid therapy. As with amphetamines, tolerance and dependence may occur.

Oral Local Anaesthetics: Certain of the local anaesthetic agents used for the treatment of cardiac arhythmias are reported to be effective in the treatment of chronic neuropathic pain. The role of these drugs in the treatment of neuropathic pain related to cancer is yet to be established and they should be regarded as second line therapy to be set aside for refractory pain. The mechanism of action is thought to be by membrane stabilisation. Drugs that have been used include mexiletine (50mg PO q8h to be increased to 800mg/d, mean dose 600mg/d), flecainide (100mg PO q12h) and tocainide (400mg PO q8h). These drugs must be used with particular caution in patients with ischaemic heart disease.

Antibiotics: The treatment of the pain of cellulitis, mucositis and fungating tumours is often greatly improved by the use of appropriate antibiotic agents.

Anaesthetic, neurolytic and neurosurgical procedures

Neural blockade, including neurosurgical procedures, can be used to block or modify the sensation of pain from the moment it is transmitted from the source to the central nervous system.

Recently the use of intraspinal opioids have greatly reduced the need for these procedures, particularly neurosurgical operations.

These procedures have to be evaluated if life expectancy is assessed to be long enough (3 months).

Local anaesthetic agents. Local anaesthetics are used for local infiltration of painful lesions and to obtain prognostic information prior to any neurolytic procedures. Side effects are primarily neurological and cardiovascular. Cardiac toxicity may occur in patients with cardiac conduction disorders or heart block. Toxicity due to elevated plasma levels may occur following injection of too large a dose, inadvertent intravenous injection or impaired metabolism of the drug itself. Local anaesthetics for epidural and spinal anaesthesia should be preservative-free in order to avoid chemical meningitis.

The addition of adrenaline counteracts the vasodilatation caused by lignocaine and prolongs the period of anaesthesia. Bupivacaine causes less vasodilatation and the addition of adrenaline does not significantly prolong the duration of anaesthesia. A simultaneous injection of a corticosteroid preparation, however, may prolong the effect of the injected local anaesthetic.

Neurolytic agents and instruments. Therapeutic nerve blocks are performed by an injection of either alcohol or phenol around the nerve, by the use of a cryoprobe or by thermocoagulation using either a laser or a radiofrequency device. All these methods produce severe neuronal damage with Wallerian degeneration, although the persistence of the basal lamina around the Schwann cell tube allows the nerves fibres to regenerate, and avoids the formation of painful neuroma. In contrast, surgical section of peripheral nerves is frequently followed by the formation of painful neuroma.

Neurolytic blocks are performed with 25–50% alcohol or 3–5% aqueous phenol. Injection of these agents will cause local tissue necrosis. Injection of alcohol causes severe pain, which is prevented if it is preceded by local anaesthetics. Cryotherapy is performed with a 2mm diameter cryoprobe cooled to about −60°; this procedure has a longer lasting effect.

Local infiltration

Neuroma. Neuroma following surgery or amputation may be treated by injection of local anaesthetic, its effect is significantly prolonged if long-acting corticosteroids are added.

Trigger point injection. Myofascial pain is characterised by local pain and tenderness in muscles, associated with pain irradiating in a non-dermatomal distribution. There are local trigger points, palpation of which produces or aggravates the symptoms; an injection with a local anaesthetic usually produces relief.

Nerve blocks

Peripheral nerve blocks may be diagnostic, prognostic or therapeutic.

Diagnostic nerve block. A temporary nerve block will determine which nerve or nerves are responsible for the patient's pain and to differentiate visceral and somatic pain. For example, a block of the stellate ganglion will abolish sympathetic pain in the upper and lower limbs.

Prognostic nerve block. A prognostic nerve block is performed to assess the adequacy of analgesia and to allow the patient to experience a gradual sensory loss and to assess the degree and severity of any motor or sphincteric disturbance.

Therapeutic nerve block. This could be temporary, prophylactic or permanent.

Temporary therapeutic nerve blocks with a local anaesthetic are used for the short term relief of severe pain before other treatments are tried. Prophylactic nerve blocks are used in situations where predictable local progression of cancer is likely to produce severe pain.

Permanent nerve blocks should only be performed after a prognostic block with a local anaesthetic. Nerve blocks are suitable for purely sensory nerves in any area as long as they do not interfere with the patient's performance status. The most frequent indication for permanent nerve blocks are the intercostal nerves where the loss of other neurological function is not clinically important; in contrast nerve blocks for the treatment of limb pain is to be avoided. The treatment may last weeks or months but its use may be sufficient when the patient is terminal.

Spinal nerve blocks. The only block performed frequently is that of intercostal nerves for chest and abdominal wall pain.

Cranial nerve blocks. The only cranial nerve block performed frequently is that of the trigeminal nerve for patients with severe pain in the anterior two-thirds of the head; block of the trigeminal nerve or Gasserian ganglion block results in good analgesia lasting for several months in about 80% of the patients. Side effects include keratosis and corneal ulceration.

Autonomic nerve blocks. Sympathetic nerve involvement produces burning pain, often with allodynia and it is usually associated with vasomotor changes (vasoconstriction, coldness, increased sweating) of the affected part and even-

tually secondary dystrophia may occur. This kind of pain responds poorly to analgesics but is resolved with local nerve blocks.

The same treatment is applied for phantom limb pain.

Stellate ganglion block. Stellate ganglion block is indicated for the relief of visceral pain associated with intrathoracic disease, sympathetic pain involving the head and neck or upper limb and for pain associated with upper limb amputation. The stellate ganglion is situated anterior to the transverse process of the seventh vertebra and incorporates all the sympathetics to the head and the neck, upper limbs and many of the intrathoracic viscera. Complications include damage to local tissues, vessels and other nerves; e.g. Horner's syndrome.

Coeliac plexus block. Coeliac plexus blocks are indicated for the treatment of severe pain in upper abdominal viscera. The coeliac plexus lies anterolateral to the body of L1. Orthostatic hypotension due to splanchnic and lower limb vasodilatation occurs frequently but usually resolves in a few days. It is more likely to occur in elderly and debilitated patients and the blood pressure should be controlled. Other complications include damage to local tissues, vessels, other nerves and diarrhoea. Relief is immediate in about 80% of patients and lasts for many months.

Lumbar sympathetic block. Lumbar sympathetic block is indicated for pain due to disease in pelvic viscera and for pain associated with lower limb amputation. Complications include hypotension and an unintentional lumbosacral plexus block, which causes weakness, and numbness of lower limbs, urinary incontinence and sexual dysfunctions.

Intraspinal nerve blocks

These involve injection of local anaesthetic or neurolytic agents into the epidural or subarachnoid space for the relief of severe pain. These are specialist techniques that require technical special skills and may cause major complications.

Local anaesthetic block. The injection of local anaesthetics into the epidural space provides excellent analgesia over several spinal segments.It can be obtained either with a single injection or by a permanent placement of a catheter in the epidural space at the desired level. The epidural catheter can be tunnelled subcutaneously and connected to a reservoir or to a continuous infusion pump. Tolerance will develop after a few days or weeks. This type of treatment is particularly useful for temporary pain relief while other kind of treatments are being organised.

Neurolytic blocks. Intraspinal neurolytic blocks involve the injection of alcohol or phenol into the epidural or subarachnoid space. The risks of these procedures are possible damage to the motor neurons producing limb weakness or paralysis as well as bladder and bowel dysfunction. The blocks are not permanent and there is a high incidence of complications such as neuralgia, painful anaesthesia, motor weakness and autonomic dysfunction.

Neurosurgical procedures

Neurosurgical procedures should be reserved for those patients with intractable pain, for whom there is no available anticancer therapy. The use of these procedures have become less common since the introduction and improvement of analgesics and other therapies.

Operations on the peripheral nerve. This operation will produce anaesthesia for a limited period and regeneration of the nerve may be complicated by the development of a painful neuroma.

Dorsal rhizotomy, or the surgical section of the sensory roots where they enter the spinal cord, may be useful in patients with severe pain limited to a few spinal segments in the trunk; it is not indicated for limb pain.

Operations on the spinal cord. Operations including dorsal entry zone lesions, anterolateral cordotomy and comissural myelotomy are specialised procedures reported to be of benefit in carefully selected patients.

Operations on the brain. Specialised neurosurgical procedures have been reported to be beneficial to a small number of highly selected patients with intractable pain. It has a very limited application to the cancer population.

Physical therapies

Physical therapy is related to the treatment of cancer pain; sometimes it is requested by the patient himself.

Mechanical therapies

Massage and exercise. Both massage and exercise, whether passive or active, relieve pain due to muscle spasm, myofascial syndromes or the general musculoskeletal discomfort associated with immobility and debility.

Manipulation. Another kind of therapy is manipulation, a commonly practised method for the treatment of pain of non-malignant origin; it is contraindicated in patients with bone metastases.

Orthotic device & mobility aids. These methods are used to reduce and prevent pain associated with movement (a walking stick can reduce weight-bearing by 25% and a crutch by as much as 45%).

Immobilisation. Patients suffering from severe pain sometimes need bed rest or a wheelchair.

Heat therapy. Heat may relieve pain as a counter-irritant stimulus by reducing the transmission of the pain stimulus in the dorsal horn of the spinal cord and may also induce inhibitory stimuli from the brain stem. The local effects of heat include muscle relaxation, increased blood flow and increased tissue compliance. It is therefore of particular benefit in the treatment of muscle spasm, myofascial pain and the general musculoskeletal discomforts associated with mobility and debility. Heat treatment may cause tissue damage and should not be used in areas where there is diminished sensation or paralysis and wherever tissues are ischaemic. It should not be used where there is infection or directly over tumour tissue. Heat can be administered by hot packs, electric heating pads, radiant heat lamps (white and infrared) and hydrotherapy. Deeper tissues may be reached via ultrasound, short wave diathermy and microwave treatment in which electromagnetic energy is converted into heat in the tissues; they should not be used near plastic prostheses or areas where bone cement has been used. These therapies do not have any special role in the treatment of cancer-related pain.

Cold therapy. Cryotherapy has the same local effects as heat therapy and the same indications; however analgesic effects last longer. It may be administered with ice massage, cold packs, or vapocoolant sprays such as ethylchloride. It should not be used in areas where there is diminished sensation, or vascular insufficiency or in patients with Raynaud's syndrome or cold hypersensitivity.

Electrical therapy

Transcutaneous electrical nerve stimulation (TENS): TENS is performed with the use of electrodes applied to the skin causing electrical activity in the large afferent fibres, taking precedence over pain signals of the spinal cord. Paraesthesia is possible in the painful area. Should conventional TENS fail, stronger electric stimulation may be used with or without needles; this treatment, operated by stimulation of the motor afferent nerves, produces muscle contraction in those muscles related to the painful area. This technique must be used with caution in patients with cancer, as strong muscle contractions may cause fractures in case of metastases; it is ineffective against visceral pain and contraindicated in patients with cardiac pacemakers. It may be effective, however, in the treatment of mild to moderate pain due to musculoskeletal disorders and neuralgia. Side effects chiefly include skin irritation. Initially there is a high response to therapy with TENS, although only a few patients obtain a long term benefit. Patients with chronic pain related to cancer rarely obtain benefit that lasts over a month, so the use of this method is very limited. In any case, if successful, it is a method that reduces the quantity of analgesics and is relatively free of complications.

Neurostimulatory treatment. Electrical stimulation of the dorsal columns of the spinal cord, the thalamus and brain centres has been reported successful for the treatment of intractable pain. It is a technique that requires surgery for electrode placement; the efficacy of the treatment in patients with pain related to advanced cancer remains to be established.

Topical counter-irritants

This method is thought to work by counter-irritation, its application stimulating neuronal activity that inhibits the passage of pain signals in the dorsal horn. Topical analgesic creams contain capsaicin and are used for post-herpetic neuralgia and arthritic pain. These creams must be applied several times a day and initially produce a burning sensation.

Acupuncture

The mechanisms by which acupuncture is used to relieve pain are not well known; its use is not uncommon in many countries today and is even officially recognised in some for the treatment of pain. Its role however in the treatment of pain related to cancer has not been defined.

Psychological and psychosocial aspects of pain control

Whilst assessing and treating the physical source of pain, the psychosocial issues must not be ignored.

Psychological, social, spiritual and cultural factors play an important role in the genesis, aggravation and improvement of pain and therefore should be taken seriously. Several members of the interdisciplinary team may be appropriate to help with these aspect of pain management.

Social, cultural and spiritual factors

Identification of these factors is of particular importance for a palliative care programme; it is necessary to consider the most appropriate interventions for each patient.

Psychological therapies

As previously described, psychological issues cannot be separated from pain in patients with advanced cancer. Various approaches are possible and controlled studies have defined the efficacy of various techniques. In any case all techniques require active patient participation and adequate training for those administering the therapies.

General psychological support. All patients with cancer must not feel abandoned. As far as is possible, patients must be involved in decisions about their care and good communication is essential in preventing unnecessary fear and anxiety. Otherwise patients are more likely to have pain and less likely to respond to the therapy.

Relaxation therapy. This kind of therapy, which has become very popular in recent years, involves a variety of techniques. The main aim of relaxation therapy is to produce general calming of the patient, which in turn helps to treat exacerbations of pain related to emotional stress. The simplest of these techniques is control of respiration.

Hypnosis. Hypnosis is claimed to be of value in the treatment of cancer-related pain and in some patients with phantom limb pain. Successful hypnosis requires that the patient has good hypnotic susceptibility and has confidence in the therapist. It may relieve anxiety and produce elevation of mood.

Biofeedback therapy. This therapy is a process in which a patient learns to control physiological responses. Electronic devices are used to detect and amplify various biological signals and convert these into signals understood by the patient. The types of biofeedback therapy used include muscle activity / tension, skin temperature, skin conduction and electroencephalography. Its role in the management of cancer-related pain remains to be established.

Operant techniques. Operant conditioning or contingency management is a method of helping patients to modify pain behaviours and related actions.

Cognitive-behavioural treatment. The aim of this treatment is to help patients identify and change their behaviour and aspects of their mood that may exacerbate pain.

Psychotherapy. Patients who suffer from anxiety, depression and emotional distress may benefit from traditional psychotherapy as well as the appropriate use of antidepressants and anxiolytic drugs. It may help patients accept the reality of their condition.

Anticancer therapy

Usually the most effective means of controlling pain is the application of anticancer therapy. The various modalities of anticancer treatment should be considered for all patients with pain. Radiotherapy is most frequently used in this situation compared to chemotherapy, although the latter when associated with hormonal therapy and surgery may be indicated in certain clinical situations.

Radiotherapy

Radiotherapy is the most effective means of controlling pain due to local tumour infiltration, however it is not a cure and its benefits must be weighed against the inconvenience it causes (e.g. transport of the patient). The purpose of radiotherapy is to kill some tumour cells, leading to a reduction of pain or other symptoms caused by the tumour itself. Naturally the efficacy of radiotherapy depends on a number of factors related to both the tumour and the radiation: more rapidly growing tumours and those with good vascular supply are naturally more sensitive to radiotherapy. Local pain caused by local tumour infiltration usually benefits from local radiotherapy, irrespective of its histology.

> The response varies with the site of the metastases: bone metastases for example are usually successful with lower doses of irradiation but the radiosensitivity of the cancer is of no importance in the treatment.

The results of radiotherapy also depend on the effective dose that can be delivered with tolerable side effects. Less favourable results are obtained when soft tissue metastases are treated, which usually require higher doses that may damage adjacent normal tissues. If possible, palliative radiotherapy should be delivered in such a way as to reduce to the minimum the side effects and the number of sessions.

Conventional radiotherapy given for tumour control involves a dose of 30–40Gy given in 10 to 20 treatment sessions over a period of 2–4 weeks; the dose given for palliative treatment is of the order of 8–20Gy given in 1–5 treatment session. Bone metastases in a limb can often be treated with a single session, whereas other areas may require multiple fractions. The response to radiotherapy is usually manifest within 2 to 4 weeks of the start of treatment, and more rapidly (a few days) with higher dose fractions. The duration is several months.

The side effects include skin reaction and inflammation of any normal tissues and mucous membranes, increased pain during first sessions due to reactive oedema.

Hemibody irradiation is also possible to the whole of the upper or lower half of the body; it has been demonstrated to offer prompt relief in a majority of patients with carcinoma of the prostate and multiple myeloma. However, the toxicity of hemibody irradiation is considerable and it should be reserved for patients with a reasonable life expectancy. Systemic administration of radioisotopes is also possible for effective pain control due to bone metastases.

Chemotherapy

The use of chemotherapy for palliative purposes depends upon the inherent chemosensitivity of the tumour; sensitive cancers include lymphoma, myeloma, leukaemia and testicular cancer. These are followed by moderately responsive tumours such as cancer of the breast, ovary and small cell carcinoma of the lung. Poorly responsive tumours are for example malignant melanoma and renal cell carcinoma.

The response to palliative chemotherapy also depends on the number and situation of the painful lesions. Chemotherapy is more likely to relieve pain due to soft tissue infiltration than to bone metastases; it is preferred to radiotherapy when there are multiple or disseminated lesions. In these cases as well, chemotherapy should be geared to produce manageable and acceptable toxicity.

Hormonal therapy

Corticoisteroids. Corticosteroids have an antitumour action and are of particular benefit for pain in patients with lymphoproliferative diseases.

Sex hormones. Patients with breast cancer respond to treatments with various hormones. The hormonal agents include tamoxifen, aminoglutethamide, progestogens, oestrogens and androgens. Patients with carcinoma of the prostate respond well to orchiectomy, oestrogens, cyproterone acetate, luteinising hormone-releasing-hormone ((LH-RH) analogues and there are improved cases of pain in patients treated with progestogens. Endometrial cancer, as well as carcinoma of the kidney, responds to progestogen therapy even though the latter has been reported to respond in only a small proportion of cases.

Surgery. Surgery is important for pain management in patients with advanced cancer. It is sometimes required for orthopaedic complications and visceral obstruction. Ablative endocrine surgery for hormone-sensitive tumours has been largely replaced by pharmacological treatment. Pain due to pathological fractures is best treated by internal surgical fixation also because it allows more rapid mobilisation and rehabilitation. The same may be said for articular prosthesis.

Pain secondary to visceral obstruction may be relieved by surgical intervention. Procedures employed include laser resection and the placement of celestin tubes for oesophageal lesions, by-pass surgery for intestinal lesions or ostomies for colonic lesions. Biliary lesions and ureteric obstruction may be relieved surgically.

Unrelieved pain

Unrelieved pain remains the fear of many patients with advanced cancer; it is still believed that the pain associated with advanced cancer does not respond to treatment. The truth is that only a very small percentage of patients (5%) have pain that is not relieved by proper treatment.

What constitutes optimal treatment does not necessarily involve the use of the latest drug, but involves the general principles of multidisciplinary palliative care. Pain must be viewed in the context of all the patient's problems.

The most frequent causes of unrelieved pain are the inadequate or improper use of analgesics: proper treatment for the relief of chronic pain requires that the appropriate drug be administered regularly, at set times and in different doses from those for acute pain. Other frequent causes for unrelieved pain may be due to problems of another kind, such as psychological, social, etc., which cause or aggravate pain. The great majority of patients with cancer can be well controlled with less than 500mg/d of parenteral morphine and requirements above this should call for an assessment for other causes of suffering. The management of these patients, despite a multidisciplinary approach, is difficult.

Pain in neonates, children and adolescents

Most children with cancer experience pain. After diagnosis, common childhood malignancies generally respond rapidly to treatment and disease-related pain often remits. If the tumour is resistant to treatment, the disease progresses rapidly, resulting in early death.

Pain in children with cancer arises more often from the treatment than from the disease. If on the one hand aggressive treatment for children increases survival rate, on the other hand it involves painful side effects (mucositis, peripheral neuropathy and infection).

The optimal treatment of a child's cancer-related pain requires an awareness, far more than in an adult, of the many factors that shape that pain. Among these are the child's developmental level, his emotional and cognitive states, his personal history, past experiences, the meaning of pain for the child, the stage of the disease, the child's fears and concerns about illness, the family's reactions and cultural background. Clinicians should be aware that children with cancer experience pain, depression, anxiety, panic, pruritus, insomnia, nausea, constipation, dyspnoea, fear of abandonment and death.

For some children, verbal communication is difficult. It is therefore of the utmost importance that the clinician should recognise the potential for pain and discomfort even if the signs are not immediately apparent.

Self-report. Methods of pain assessment can be different: the self-report can be used for children over the age of 4. Answers can be verbal or non-verbal. Often children will not respond to questions verbally, especially if they are anxious or depressed or are experiencing severe pain. Some investigators have used drawings as a rating scale for younger children, whereas for those over the age of 5 who can understand the concepts of order and number they prefer a numerical rating scale or a VAS. To determine the location of pain, children can be asked either to point to their body or use a body map. Children over the age of 4 can use colouring pencils to locate pain on a body map.

Behavioural observation. Behavioural observation is the primary assessment approach for non-verbal children and is an additional assessment for verbal children. Observations should take into consideration vocalisations, verbalisations, facial expressions, muscle tension and rigidity, guarding of body parts, temperament, activity and general appearance. It must also take into account the voluntary expression of pain, the direct signs of pain and psychomotor atonia.

Observations are problematic in that the stimulus for behaviours or changes is not always clear. For example, children cry in response to pain, as well as fear, loneliness and overstimulation. Clinicians may misinterpret behaviours such as sleeping, watching television and using humour as the absence of pain when, in fact, the child is attempting to control pain. Infants may become apathetic and refuse communication after only a few days of continuous severe pain, and suffering experienced by older children with cancer may blunt behaviours and is a source of pain. Other factors that inhibit behavioural responses include intubation, use of sedatives, the final phases of the illness, weakness and depression. Therefore, the use of behavioural observation is very useful for guidelines but requires close attention to the context.

Pain management

Pain management for children cannot be considered without consultation with the parents and the treatment should be in conformity with their beliefs and preferences.

Medical interventions. Medical interventions include the use of analgesics, adjuvant agents, palliative chemotherapy, radiation therapy, neurosurgical approaches. In most cases analgesics alone are enough to provide adequate pain relief. Occasionally regional analgesia is beneficial.

Analgesics and adjuvants. Acetaminophen and NSAIDs are useful for mild to moderate pain. The rectal route is preferable for children who cannot take medication orally; it must be said, however, that children do not like this route and may refuse to take the medication. Rectal administration is contraindicated for children who are neutropenic or thrombocytopenic and for those with mucositis. These contraindications and the irregular absorption of the rectal route limit its usefulness in the treatment of severe pain. Because children with cancer are often thrombocytopenic, NSAIDs are contraindicated. Their use, however, provides excellent results for those children who are not at risk.

The administration of Acetaminophen and NSAIDs varies according to the intensity of the pain: for mild pain, as-needed administration is appropriate, otherwise around-the-clock administration is necessary.

Opioid analgesics. For moderate to severe pain, opioid analgesics are recommended. Studies of the risks of addiction in children have not been done but studies of survivors of childhood cancer report history of severe unhealed pain.

Route of administration. Whenever possible opioids are to be administered orally, the liquid form or suspension is the best form. Parenteral administration is indicated when:

- the child cannot take medication by mouth, for reasons such as nausea, vomiting, obstruction and mucositis;

- absorption may be compromised;
- the pain is severe and requires a rapid titration to effect;
- frequent and severe breakthrough or incident-related pain occurs;
- the oral route requires frequent administration of medication or large numbers of pills. Intramuscular injections are to be avoided because they are painful and frightening to children.

Severe pain is an emergency requiring careful assessment. The initial dose of opioid administration for children is 1 mg/kg/d orally; intervals between administrations are the same as for adults. Continuous infusion of morphine, at a starting dose of 0.02 to 0.04 mg/kg per hour for children over 6 months of age has been well studied.

Continuous infusion is indicated when intermittent doses:

- cause undue somnolence at the time of peak effect;
- provide inadequate analgesia at the usual starting doses;
- must be administered more frequently; the process for dose increase and titration to effect is the same as in adults.

Agent. Morphine is the preferred starting drug for severe pain; codeine and oxycodone can be used for moderate pain. Meperidine should be used only in exceptional circumstances such as hypersensitivity to morphine and other drugs, and side effects are prevented by the use of anticonvulsants.

Patient-Controlled Analgesia (PCA). PCA can be used in children over 5 years of age. Even in children, regular assessment of their vital signs and level of consciousness is necessary when p-arenteral opioids are used.

Side effects. Young children have difficulty in communicating subjective symptoms such as nausea, pruritus, constipation and dysphoria; the preverbal child may only show generalised discomfort.

One of the most feared but exceptional side effects of opioid use is respiratory depression. The initial dose of naloxone in children is 2 mcg/kg, to be repeated every minute, it should be titrated gradually until the patient resumes adequate respiratory effort.

Adjuvants. Tryciclic antidepressants can be used in the same way as for adults. Generally the starting dose is low (0.2 mg/kg of amitriptyline) and then increased to about 1–2 mg/kg daily. Care should be taken in children who have received large doses of cardiotoxic anthracyclines. Stimulants such as dextroamphetamine can also be used at a starting dose of 0.05 mg/kg to be increased gradually.

Analgesics for neonates and young children

Paracetamol can also be administered to increase analgesia. The use of opioids requires special consideration and expertise. Young infants, especially premature babies or those who have neurologic abnormalities or pulmonary disease, are susceptible to respiratory depression when systemic opioids are used. The infant's metabolism is altered so that the elimination half-life is longer and the blood-brain barrier is more permeable. Intensive monitoring is advisable up to about 1 year of age for non-ventilated infants who are receiving opioids, because extreme sedation and reduced respiratory effort may be difficult to assess.

Respiratory depression is anyhow dose related; the initial dose for infants under 6 months should be about one-quarter to one-third of the dose recommended for older infants. The usual effective dosage is 60–80 mg/kg/d.

Epidural analgesia. The use of epidural analgesia is appropriate when systemically administered analgesics do not achieve pain control and cause unacceptable side effects. The maximum recommended dose is 0.4 mg/kg for bupicacaine and 2 mg/kg for lidocaine.

Epidural infusions that exceed the recommended rates may cause convulsions. Expertise and close monitoring is necessary.

Non pharmacologic methods

Non pharmacologic methods used by adults may be adapted for children. Preparation for painful events needs a distraction technique, which could involve the use of a puppet, a favourite cartoon character or an animal. When a child is in pain, the presence of a parent is usually helpful. Other methods of psychological support include relaxation or use of imagery, being picked up or changing positions, simple interventions that have powerful effects. Although not well researched in children, methods such as physical therapy, TENS, hot and cold packs, etc. may be of help to relieve pain.

Assessment of pain management strategies

The most important consideration to be made in the assessment of pain management in children with cancer is developmental issues and problems that affect the family's integrity.

Elderly patients

Elderly patients are often undertreated because a certain amount of pain is considered part of normal aging, either because it is badly assessed or because of mistaken beliefs about their pain sensitivity, pain tolerance and ability to use opioids. Elderly patients, like other adults, require aggressive pain assessment. Studies on the elderly are very few and this category of patient is most likely to be excluded from certain therapies such as rehabilitation programmes. It has been estimated that the prevalence of pain in those over 65 is double compared with the adult population.

Elderly patients with cancer often have other chronic diseases, such as cognitive impairment, delirium and dementia, which pose serious obstacles to pain assessment, and often pain assessment instruments in such cases are useless. This suggests that the elderly require far more frequent pain assessment than patients of other age groups; in some cases behavioural observation is required.

NSAIDs are very effective whether alone or associated with opioids for pain management; in the elderly, however, there is a risk of gastric and renal toxicity and further factors that may contribute to other side effects include multiple medical diagnoses with multiple drug interactions. To protect the gastric mucosa for example, the administration of misoprostol in association with NSAIDs would be beneficial.

Elderly patients benefit from opioids but it must be kept in mind that they are subject to Cheyne-Stokes respiratory patterns particularly during sleep. The elderly tend to be more sensitive to the analgesic effects of opioids, which seem to have a longer duration of pain relief. They also tend to be more sensitive to sedation and respiratory depression, probably as a result of alterations in metabolism and in the distribution and excretion of the drugs. For this reason, the prolonged use of longer-acting drugs such as methadone requires caution.

Elderly people generally have a reduced glomerular filtration rate. Opioids produce cognitive and neuropsychiatric dysfuntion through poorly defined mechanisms that, in part, include the accumulation of active metabolites such as morphine-6-glucuronide or normeperidine. Opioid dose titration should take into account not only analgesic effects but also side effects that extend beyond cognitive impairment. Other side effects include urinary retention (a threat in elderly males with prostatic hyperplasia), constipation and intestinal obstruction or respiratory depression.

Local anaesthetic infusions may result in cognitive impairment if significant drug levels in the blood are reached. Orthostatic hypotension may result from tricyclic antidepressant administration: precautions should be taken during ambulation.